T0148417

Wouldn't It Be Nice If...

You Could Be Healthy on a Budget

A Really Simple Guide to Health for Really Busy People

Stephanie S. Lalosh

Order this book online at www.trafford.com
or email orders@trafford.com

Most Trafford titles are also available at major online book retailers.

Printed in the United States of America.

ISBN: 978-1-4269-7623-0 (sc)
ISBN: 978-1-4269-7626-1 (e)

Library of Congress Control Number: 2011912371

Trafford rev. 07/16/2011

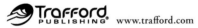 www.trafford.com

North America & international
toll-free: 1 888 232 4444 (USA & Canada)
phone: 250 383 6864 ♦ fax: 812 355 4082

For the Renz girls.

Clara, Roberta, and especially Patsy, who always
wanted an author in the family.

Preface

Keeping It Simple, Keeping It Healthy, Keeping It *Real*

It's funny how things never quite turn out how one might expect. This book is a prime example. I thought I was going to help my fiancé create ads and flyers for advertisements so that he could begin consulting with people who wanted to get and live healthy. Unsure of exactly how or where we would start, we began drafting topics that we felt would benefit those seeking his help. Within a month of discussing health topics, we were drafting a book. Who knew?

I know not everyone thinks like me, but one of my favorite words in life is "efficient." We all have busy lifestyles, so who can afford not to be? So, even if many others don't think like me, I am sure they can all relate to the need for efficiency, and that really is one of the main objectives of this book. I've seen the ones that list *volumes* of resources, which are wonderful, and my fiancé really loves. However, that isn't always "functional" for me. (That's another of my favorite words.) I find that I just don't have time to try everything on the list! But…if I understand the "how" and the "why" about products and procedures and what they do, I can really make a better decision about what will be most effective, and efficient for me. So, as far as this working relationship between me and my fiancé goes, our deal works like this: he spits out information and details, and I turn them into a narrative that people can comprehend and relate to. Fair enough. Funny, that's pretty much how we continue to handle health topics in our own life. Ultimately all we want to do is to reach out to people, in whatever way, shape, or form that may be, and let them know that if we can do it, anyone can do it. Consequently, we are both now accomplishing what we most desire to do, and we hope you will find that you are able to take something away from this book that will ultimately help you get started on and continue your own path to a healthier lifestyle.

TABLE OF CONTENTS

INTRODUCTION

$\mathcal{B}$eing healthy. Who doesn't want to be? My experience has been that no one truly desires to be *un*healthy. So, why do so many people wait to start to get healthy? Why don't more people make being healthy a part of their lifestyle? My observations have helped me to come to some of my own conclusions. After talking with others and observing carefully, I have found a few common barriers, both physical and mental. I've learned that if you just take a look, you can always find a starting point. For some, it may be diet and some light exercise, while for others it may be necessary to get healthier in the mind in order to get motivated and realize it can be done. I have always made health and fitness a priority in my life, and yet I have also encountered what are probably the most common physical and mental "roadblocks": thinking it is not affordable and not knowing how or where to start. How can one navigate his way through the plethora of information and have any idea where to start? The answer to that problem is *simple*. Start anywhere. Start somewhere. This book is a result of trying to help people overcome those feelings that prohibit them from getting started on a healthy path. I too have felt overwhelmed by the amount of information regarding health and wellness (which I still love to read about) but I have been fortunate to have a fiancé who has been able to simplify concepts for me and therefore deepen my understanding. As I continue to learn and understand how and why things work, I have been able to "design" a healthy lifestyle that fits my personality, needs, schedule, and budget. My fiancé has done the same. Even though we both include certain routines into our day, we both also find that we need to adapt aspects of our health regimen to our personalities and schedules, and therefore do differ in some aspects.

As a teacher, I interact every day with adults and students alike that have so many questions regarding health, and, while I am not a doctor, and can not advise them medically, I can share with them my experiences as an individual and also the experiences my fiancé and I have had in trying to raise a healthy family. My students especially are full of questions. While answering these questions is always a pleasure, (as this is easily my favorite discussion topic) we felt that we needed a way to reach out to, and more importantly, to *help* more people get on the road to being healthy. This simple, real book is our way of doing what we enjoy most: helping people to be healthy, simply, and affordably. We have tried to keep it simple and real by explaining concepts and not prescribing a program. We hope that understanding how and why things work will help you take ownership of and design your own healthy lifestyle. Read it the old-fashioned way (beginning at page one) or start in the middle, or start at the end. Start wherever makes sense for *YOU*. We designed the book simply so that it's easy to decide what works best for you.

Yes, there are some things that we all need to do to be healthy, but we all have individual needs as well. Ask yourself, "Which one of these areas will give me the boost that I need to accomplish the others?" and start there. It's amazing how much you will want to continue once you start. We know you will because being healthy feels *good*. Being healthy is manageable *and* affordable. However, nothing is for free, and by free we are not always referring to monetary matters. Part of the journey down a healthy path requires being willing to try some new things, and to work through some difficulties. As you read the book, we'll also share our own experiences with you about our own attempts to navigate our way through a healthy lifestyle (just so you know you are not alone if things don't go quite as you expect initially), and our continued efforts to find new, better, healthier, and even simpler and more affordable ways to continue a healthy lifestyle for us and for our children (while both trying to work full-time). It hasn't always been easy, but because being healthy feels *good*, we persevere.

THE BODY

A healthy body. We all have different ideas about what a healthy body is. Does it mean skinny? Does it mean muscular? Does it mean more about what's happening on the inside? I have come to the conclusion that it is a combination of things, and my perceptions of what is healthy have changed considerably as I have learned about and experienced new and better ways of being healthy. Let me first address some of that nasty controversy about why what's on the outside matters. Growing up with a 5' 9" frame, I always maintained what all the magazines and doctors' charts said was a healthy weight for me. It might have been about 145-150 pounds. I played three varsity sports, and ate fairly healthy, although not perfectly. So, I thought nothing of the size 10 that I wore consistently, and was even more proud, when, after my second child, I was still wearing it! I had always been told I was "skinny" and never thought it a possibility that I would ever wear a smaller size. I thought that genetically this is what I had been dealt, and, in fact, I found it "vain" to consider wearing a smaller size. Exercise has always been a focal point in my life, so if I was exercising and still wearing that size 10, that must be what I could expect for the rest of my life, right? Wrong!

Fast forward three years later…I weigh 135 pounds and wear a healthy size 2/4. I learned how to tackle the number one health problem in my life, and in the lives of everyone. More importantly, I realize that a focus on my weight, muscle tone, and fat percentage is NOT about vanity…this really is about being healthy and about maintaining my health for my children's sake as well, and it scares me a little that it took me until my 30's to become aware of and to start tackling the biggest problem facing us all. While I do strongly feel that we should love our loved ones for who they are, I am also a firm believer that we should help them to be healthy *because* we love them. The "outside," as you will see, is, in many ways, a reflection of (although not ultimately a predictor of) how healthy we and our loved ones are, and therefore we should want to see positive physical changes in both.

The Problem

The problem really can be summed up in one word: *toxicity*. Therefore the solution can also be summed up on one word: ***detoxify***. Remove toxicity, and we will see many positive changes in our health and in our lives. And, by the way, the issue of toxicity will be the common denominator that ties this book together. It truly does affect all of the other domains of our lives. But, let's get back to the issue in regard to creating a healthy body. We live in a toxic world, and that is the real and simple truth. We need to find ways to minimize toxicity within ourselves in order to be healthy, but first, we need to know where these toxins that are bombarding us are coming from.

This bulleted list is simple, and maybe a little scary, but rest assured you can find solutions.

- our food
- our air
- our personal care products
- our cleaning / air-freshening products
- our cell phones, TV's, and other electronic devices
- our sleeping habits
- our doctor/dental visits

Does this mean we avoid all of this "stuff" at all costs? Of course not. We are here, as real people, who aren't doctors, researchers, or scientists to try to share our experiences about how we have worked and are still working to find ways to eliminate or reduce toxicity to its lowest terms in all of these areas. Since I am an English teacher, I would like to present you with an analogy to help illustrate the importance of a clean liver in regard to the issue of toxicity. (Keep in mind that your liver burns your FAT!)

> Toxins plug your liver the same way that an air filter in your car or your oil filter becomes "plugged." I'm sure most of you make sure that these are always clean, and that your car if therefore burning fuel (food) as efficiently as possible, right? You also try to maintain your vehicle so that it lasts you long-term, and has fewer "repair bills" down the road, correct? So, why not do the same with your body? If you want your liver to burn fat, process food, and filter your blood efficiently, it must be clean...and, just like your car, investing a little extra to maintain it

now may save you "maintenance" costs down the
road.

Why does this matter? The answer is, again, simple. **Fat cells store
toxins**. Toxins cause diseases like cancer. They are also the cause of
many aches and pains that we have, which commonly get diagnosed
as "arthritis," "bursitis," "tendonitis," and many other things. We
are just too toxic! If we do not have fat cells to store those toxins,
we significantly reduce our chances of developing a disease like
cancer, and increase our chances of getting rid of the pain! While
some of us may be genetically predisposed to some of these issues,
we can work to prevent them from actually rearing their ugly heads
by not providing the tools necessary to do so. Still think removing
fat is just about vanity? I'll share a personal tragedy with you. This
is a particularly trenchant issue for me, having lost two aunts (one
age 39, and one age 56) and a grandmother to cancer. Having
watched their struggles, and the toll it took on my many other
family members helping to care for them, I know that I do not ever
want my children to have the burden of caring for me, and I do not
want them to have to endure the pain and suffering of battling the
disease. Even further, I can't imagine how my cousins managed to
keep going after losing their mother at the tender ages of 10 and 14.
So, **keep your liver clean**! Help it to burn fat efficiently. And, by
the way, (ladies) fat cells only grow as toxins fill them…they also
shrink when there is less there to fill them. So, no, we don't need to
have cellulite, and we CAN get rid of it! Hooray!

*In case you are interested, I dropped **two dress
sizes** when I started to detoxify by buying the

organic version of everything I was eating! (And I didn't eat anything with white sugar or high-fructose corn syrup.) No extra exercise necessary, and, "Hello size 6!" Now I really thought I'd never be smaller, but, as you know, this story has an even happier ending than a size 6.

Our Solutions

Our food: Eat as much organic food as possible! Which, as you will see, may require you to eat less! How's that for weight loss? I always feel the need to clarify the definition of organic food. Most of my high school English students think that organic means "tastes bad," "whole-grain," and "gross!" when, in fact, it means "full of nutrients," "tastes great," **"toxin-free,"** and "simply healthy!" (Thanks RCS Class of 2011, for helping to inspire this book.) Organic food is simply food that is grown, produced, or raised without the use of chemicals, chemical fertilizers, hormones, antibiotics, artificial flavors, sweeteners, and/or other foreign substances that the body should not be ingesting, and the liver should not have to process. Further, it is important to understand that the body feels "full" when it has sufficient nutrients. Organic products are much more chock-full of nutrients than traditional products, so we can actually eat less and still get what we need! Remember, meat and fish are included in this! Fish should be wild caught, while meat and milk should be hormone and antibiotic-free, and ideally grass-fed (or from grass-fed cows). We'll offer assistance with this in Part 6.

"Going organic" is an area in which I have the most concerns expressed to me by people trying to make ends meet every month, while still trying to give their children the best start possible. Next to the cost, the most common concern is being able to locate the desired organic products. We prefer to buy all of our groceries in organic form, and in order to do so we have to cut costs in other areas, as well as really think about what products we are actually buying. Think about how much one might spend on junk such as soda, chips, etc. Eliminating those purchases and applying that money to the cost of the organic products is one way to start pulling together some extra dollars to make your organic purchases. Joining a food co-op can also be a great way to make organic more affordable, and it supports a great cause.

"But I don't buy that stuff!" Being a "health nut," I wasn't making those soda and chip purchases either, so I had to think about other ways that I could cut a few items from my list to get the things that I really needed for me and my family. One technique I have also tried is to buy organic ingredients and cook or bake the treats my family wants, rather than buy the finished product in organic form.

If this still seems overwhelming, try to prioritize your organic purchases. The best way we can think of to help you to prioritize is to have you think of what you consume the MOST of in your home. While I am sure there will be a few basic items that most households have in common, this will be an area in which you are adapting a healthy lifestyle to you. Whatever you consume the MOST of, purchase in organic form. (A list of products that should be a priority in organic form is provided in Part 6.)

You may have to check a few different stores in order to find the best price on your organic items, but, we promise, it will be worth it. It took me a few months of comparison shopping, but I now know which stores to go to in order to get the best price on our organic, and most essential items. And, yes, I do have to make several stops when shopping, but I try to hit a store or two around orthodontist visits, sports, and vehicle maintenance. Schedule-juggling is a fact of life for all moms, so don't beat yourself up if it takes a little time to fall into a system. It will come! It is also important to avoid several things. Here are some foods (if you can call it food) we avoid at all costs:

- white sugar
- high-fructose corn syrup
- anything processed
- soy products

So, now that you are fueling your body with "premium," how do you maximize your gas milage? Again, the answer is simple: **detoxing.** Flip through a few pieces of health literature, and you will discover cleanse, after cleanse, after cleanse, many of which are of very good quality. Cleanses for just about any purpose can be purchased in stores and on-line, and range from inexpensive to hundreds of dollars. These include the Be Pure, McCombs, and other cleanses recommended by Kevin Trudeau. Some programs even have payment plans. This is one area in which we have tried to customize our health program. Rather than spending hundreds of dollars on cleanses, we use the money to purchase our organic food, and instead use a much more affordable, and highly effective system. This old-time remedy has been around for years, so if it's not broken, don't fix it, right! (Now I know why my grandmother gave this to my mom and 10 other aunts and uncles.) We'll let you in on the secret momentarily.

We need to get toxins out of ALL of our cells (in addition to our livers) to remove the tools that any other genetic predispositions may need to manifest themselves. This requires a team effort between your cells and your liver, and we have learned to accomplish this with a combination of eating raw foods, juicing, using coffee enemas, and taking castor oil. While individually these are all great, they are most effective when used in conjunction with each other. The nutrients in raw foods and juice will get into cells and force toxins from them, but will not necessarily flush all of them from your body via its normal elimination mechanisms. The coffee enemas and castor oil will flush out toxins they can access, but need the juice and raw foods to flush the toxins to places where the enemas and castor oil can get to them…mainly through the liver.

It is important to understand how the castor oil process works to illustrate why this is so effective. Again, the English teacher in me feels that an analogy is most helpful in visualizing this process.

> Think of a dam. Dams are built for safety, to protect, to conserve and preserve. If they give, disaster strikes. Your liver does this for your body. It is holding back poisonous toxins so that your bloodstream is not polluted. The castor oil process helps to relieve some of the "work" that the dam must do. Even our local dam is being reinforced due to years of use, wear, tear, and lack of up-keep. Imagine what would happen if it burst? As for the

castor oil…try to picture your liver opening up, and releasing a flow of toxins…almost like some dams do. In this case, however, the release is a controlled process preserving both the dam (your liver) and everything it is supposed to protect.

The beauty of cleansing with castor oil is that as it travels it takes toxins with it from the esophagus, from the stomach, and right through the intestines, while along the way stimulating the liver to release accumulated toxins via the bile duct. The castor oil will take a good amount of the toxins out; however, we are continuously re-accumulating toxins into our bodies just by living in this modern world. Furthermore, because many of us are just coming to the realization that we need to get healthy, we need to make up for lost time. As a population, we have become so toxic over the years that just one castor oil cleanse will not suffice. We started our process by juicing daily and taking castor oil one to two times per month. We have since modified the frequency of our cleansing program to fit our needs, lifestyles, and, yes our personalities! No matter what your schedule, always be sure that you have adequately nutrified yourself via juice and raw food if you want to cleanse with castor oil more frequently. (By the way, a bottle of it only costs me $2.76 in Walmart).

If this sounds like a good fit for you, or you just want to read a funny story, then you will want to continue reading here. If not, jump down to juicing! But, really, you don't want to miss this. I'll share my experience with cleansing with castor oil. The beginning was really rough for *me*, but *my mom* sailed right through hers, so it's hard to predict how the first few months will go. (I think she had the advantage of having to take it as a child, because she downs it like a champ).

I started by taking two tablespoons and following it with a cup of coffee. (My fiancé's instructions). It occurred to me months later that I was not drinking organic coffee, though. That's the reality… so many little details that you realize you miss along the way. It happens! Just move on and do your best to fix it. (I bought some organic coffee). Dark roast is preferable. Take it before bed, as your body starts its natural cleansing process and works through the night anyway. You will want to make sure you are at home, trust me! Even if the body didn't naturally cleanse at night, which it does, I would **highly** suggest you do it at night when you are home anyway! You might even want to get a babysitter- seriously. After changing my frequency of consumption, I did further adapt this process, and my fiancé and I continue to share ideas about how to make it work for us and our bodies.

I made a few other changes to my initial procedure as well. I found I did not like the dark roast coffee, so I switched to medium roast, but I really didn't like that either, so I just stopped following it with coffee. The castor oil still works without it, but the coffee makes the "cleansing" faster when I drink it. My mom uses tea afterward. You will need to individualize this process for you. My fiancé and I also find that having a few crackers or a little cookie right after helps with the after-taste. We've experimented, and found that you really can choose to "chase" it with just about anything that works for you, whether it is food or drink.

Keep in mind that everyone reacts differently. My first reaction to this process was very intense, which had me doubled over, and sent my fiancé into hysterical laughter. (Significant others- just so you know, this first time reaction isn't funny! Be supportive! When it's over we can all laugh). A pretty intense "healing crisis" happened to me, but not to my mom. My mom's was less intense. We think the difference may be because I was already juicing and therefore flushing toxins out of my cells (carried via my blood stream) to my liver. Basically, as I just stated, I had already been forcing a lot of toxins to my liver to be processed. The castor oil relieved my liver's "toxic load," and, as the toxins exit, the body can often react with slight fever or nausea. The good news is that it was only this one time that I had a reaction like that, and it got better every time.

I cleansed on weekends only at first because I felt fatigued afterward. Now, however, after more than a year of following this process, I wake up feeling like a million bucks, and full of energy! I rock my workouts on these mornings. While I don't look forward to actually taking the castor oil (who would?), I look forward to castor oil nights, knowing how awesome I will feel the next day, how far I've come, and that my fiancé can't amuse himself at my expense anymore! Remember, we mentioned that nothing is for free, and you have to be willing to work through some things.

Let's take a second and think back to the oil filter analogy. If given only one choice of maintenance for your vehicle, wouldn't it most likely be regularly cleaning and maintaining the oil and oil filter? The same holds true for your liver. If you were to ignore all the other healthy suggestions in this book, and focus solely on taking two tablespoons of castor oil one time per month, you would find yourself an infinitely healthier person, just as your vehicle will run much more efficiently with regular cleansing. This is why we have placed this discussion so near the top of our list. It is affordable and effective. Castor oil. An oldie, but a "goodie." Ooooh...maybe "effective" is a better word.

Now on to my favorite part of our solution- juicing. We've already explained the fact that the nutrients, vitamins, and minerals from juice and raw food push their way into all cells of the body, and force toxins out to be eliminated via our helpful cleansing processes. I use a pound of organic carrots, and one organic granny smith apple. I just pick that apple for the taste. Any organic apple will do. I try to get at least 16 ounces of juice a day. This gets me the most "bang for my buck," so to speak. After all, I am living on a teacher's salary! However, don't limit your sights to only juicing carrots and apples if you can afford it. You can juice just about anything and it is wonderful. Juice your greens, chards, and other fruits and veggies. Make sure you keep them organic. If you can grow your own, even better, and use the pulp as compost. The idea is that you are getting all the nutrients from a lot more fruits and veggies than you could probably eat in a day.

When considering cost, it is important to **choose your juicer carefully**! All are not created equal. You want to make sure that consider several criteria, and you can compare juicers online. I used www.discountjuicers.com. "You must choose, but choose wisely." In order to understand why it is necessary to choose wisely, it is important to understand the other benefits of juicing. This may sound too much like Indiana Jones, but, hey, juicing is probably the next best thing to the fountain of eternal youth. In addition to vitamins, etc., fresh juice provides the body with enzymes. This is important because, for most of us, our digestive systems are not firing on all cylinders due to imbalances caused by years of taking antibiotics. Therefore, we do not digest efficiently, and food sits in our intestines and produces toxins that our body absorbs. What a vicious cycle! We will discuss helpful solutions for this issue later, but it is important to understand the need to get these essential enzymes from your juice. Enzymes are responsible for catalyzing (enhancing the speed/efficiency) of every chemical reaction that occurs on a cellular level. Heat destroys the essential enzymes. Further, juice must be consumed within three hours of juicing, or the enzymes break down due to oxygen exposure. That's after it is pressed, by the way. My fiancé taught me this snazzy little trick for when I am in a time crunch, trying to get out of the house with two children in the morning: if I grind the fruits at night, I can cover it and then press it in the morning. It's little tricks like this that you will discover and will make all the difference in finding a way to fit it all in.

So, I mentioned earlier that there are a few criteria you want to consider when purchasing a juicer. The best juicers make juicing a two-step process: grinding the fruits and/or veggies, and then pressing the juice out from the pulp. This also tends to produce the largest yield. Further, a juicer should not spin too quickly, or it will heat up and kill enzymes, it should not produce a lot of foam, which, the two-step juicers with a press will not do, and it should grind the fruits and veggies properly. So, compare juicers on-line, and remember that this is an investment in your future. This is one area where you will want to invest some money, as it should be a long-term investment. My juicer came with a 10-year warranty, and grinds slowly with an auger and doesn't get hot. (The ones that spin fast often produce too much heat). There are other styles with even better warranties than mine, but at about $350, I've been thrilled with the amount that it yields and the quality of the juice it gives me. If I had my "d'ruthers," I would personally purchase a top-of-the-line Norwalk juicer at www.norwalkjuicers.com, as recommended by Dr. Gerson, who is known for curing cancer through organic food, juices and detoxification.

Remember also to not neglect the importance of eating RAW FOOD! The enzymes and fiber in raw food are essential for health, and help the food to digest itself. (We've already discussed why this matters). It's like eating with no penalty! The calories take care of themselves. Raw, organic fruits and veggies are also full of the nutrients your body needs to flush toxins from cells. We have provided a list at the end of this book to help you determine which raw foods it is most critical to purchase in organic form. Following this list will help when making decisions in a tight grocery budget.

My six-year old daughter would tell me there is an "AB" pattern happening here. We talked first about nutrifying (organic food), then cleansing (castor oil), then nutrifying (juicing), so guess what's next! That's right, cleansing! Here we present you with another method that we have found affordable and manageable. Again, the choice is yours to make about what works, and since variety is the spice of life, we feel that the more options people have, the more likely they are to be successful due to the fact that they have choice in how to go about accomplishing goals. (Research shows that students are more successful in school when given choice, so it makes sense that the same concept would apply to helping people create a desired lifestyle).

Another option available to help cleanse the body is the coffee enema. The coffee enema is designed to work a little differently from the castor oil, but offers most of the same benefits. This procedure is a fundamental part of Dr. Gerson's natural cancer cures as well, and is, as it sounds, literally, an enema that utilizes coffee to cleanse. Organic, of course, and preferably dark roast. The caffeine from the coffee is absorbed from the large intestine, and taken to the liver via the portal vein. This, like the castor oil, opens the bile ducts in the liver, just like the dam analogy I gave you earlier.

In order to use this cleanse, you will need at least 12-15 minutes of "private time," as near to the bathroom as possible. One of the differences in this procedure from taking the castor oil is that you will need to hold the enema, hence, the required "private time." Holding the enema will actually increase the liver's ability to detoxify your blood by 600-700%! Taken rectally, you will then need to lie on your right side and draw your knees to your chest. Breathe through the nose and out the mouth. Don't panic if you can't hold for the full 12-15 minutes. You will work up to it if it doesn't come immediately. If you feel that this may be the system for you, a more detailed explanation of the procedure, and instructions for preparing the coffee are available at www.gerson.org.

Back to nutrifying! One more step that we have decided to add to our daily health regimen is to take supplements. Many vitamins and minerals can be supplied by a quality diet, but we feel that for us, taking a few extras is something that we need to do for us, and for our children. After all, what are the odds of getting them to take castor oil the way I do? Probably slim to none. All of our children have very different eating habits, regardless of what kind of diet they have been raised on. Therefore, there are a few common supplements we give to them all. We make sure that they have the following:

- Silverhydrosol- this ionized silver supplement does wonders for the immune system without building up in the body, and has significantly reduced school absences in our children. It also tastes like water, so they look forward to taking it. This amazing product is available online at www.helpingamericatogether.com.

- Zeolytes- available on the same website, these minerals reduce the amount of heavy metals in the body, and with one child in orthodontics these drops have been very helpful in helping to reduce the amount of heavy metals in the body. Although black in color, these, again, taste like water, and go down easily!

We also individualize their and our daily supplement routine. In addition to maintaining health, we have found that other supplements can prevent many other issues such as allergies. Some of the supplements that we have found it a priority to provide to us all (whether it be in pill form or powder in smoothie) include the following:

- MSM-in addition to helping with allergies, this helps us with pain, inflammation, and joint health. This is also available in pill or powder form.

- Vitamin C

- Iodine-Kelp is a whole food supplement that provides iodine and many other trace minerals that the body needs. Lugol's solution is simply iodine, and is highly absorbable. Since iodine is essential for thyroid health, either one of these methods of getting the iodine you need is great.

- Coral Calcium
- Vitamin D3 in the winter months (since we aren't getting as much sun).
- Coconut Oil-it took us a while, but we found it in pill form! Talk about a celebration. We tried melting it and taking 2 tablespoons, and although it is funny to look back on, it sure wasn't funny trying to get it down when we first started! Trust me, it's too hot to drink when melted, and chunks up quickly if you try to put it in anything cooler to try to drink it down. I would prefer to not think about how I know that. Coconut oil is preferable over fish oil, as it offers all of the same benefits as fish oil (omega-3, etc.), but without the risk of pollutants that fish may ingest from polluted waters.

We have found that in addition to detoxifying, remaining proactive is essential to a healthy lifestyle. Again, you need to find what works for you, and, of course, determine what your greatest health needs are. There are supplements available in catalogs, department stores, health food stores, on-line, and just about anywhere else that you can think of. We have found that we get good prices and reasonable shipping via Swanson vitamins. However, look around and find what you need at the best price to make it work for you.

Looks like we are back to detoxing. This time we have a little twist on the subject. The subject of this "detoxification" is not of removal, but of limitation to exposure. Unfortunately, this next issue is going to be a very real issue that is difficult to avoid, and therefore merits its own discussion. One of the largest pollutants of our bodies is electromagnetic radiation, which we need to be very careful to limit. We've all heard that cell phones can cause brain cancer and other complications. Did you know that you can actually purchase filters for your phone to block those electromagnetic waves?

While most of us may be conscious of the dangers of cell phones, are we conscious of the frequencies we are getting from your hi-def TV's and computers? Who knows what I am being bombarded with as I type this book? There are other items that can be purchased to help us to filter out those frequencies so that they are not harmful. In addition, we can try doing a few things the old-fashioned way. Read a BOOK instead of holding a kindle. It is amazing what holding a real book can do for us in addition to reducing radiation. People are physical beings, and therefore need to interact with the physical world and therefore stimulate our nervous system. Our bodies receive feedback through touch, and holding a book allows us to do that instead of reading from a screen shooting frequencies at us. Talk about being an easy target!

Too many children and adults are now spending too much time in a "virtual" reality and interaction with physical matter is decreasing significantly as time goes on. Think about the number of children having difficulty concentrating in school. Those precious little brains are developing around EMR and immediate feedback, which is still not the standard method of teaching in school. We need to get our children off the electronics, and out in the fresh air. Parenting is more difficult than it has ever been, and getting children outside to play and to be physical is difficult in tight schedules. It is easy to let the TV or computer "give us a hand" as we try to cook dinner, clean the house, and do a myriad of other things. Believe me, I know! However, it is imperative that we get our children and **ourselves** back out into nature to maintain our balance.

Let's finish this pattern with a bang! How cool would it be if you could fortify your cells *and* detox at the same time? Guess what, you can! One of my personal favorites in the steps necessary to both nutrify and detoxify is exercise. Do I have days I don't want to? Sure. We all do. But the bottom line is that exercise helps fortify our cells with oxygen, and sweat helps us pump out toxins from our bodies. Since I can't afford to build a sauna in my home, or to purchase an infra-red portable sauna, I have found that sweating from exercise is the next best thing. And, this at least keeps me looking toned, healthy, young, and wearing my new size.

The bottom line is that any movement is better than no movement, but some movements are better than others, and believe me, I have tried lots. We all have different body types, so different things will work for all of us, but I know that I need, and the average person really needs to sweat for atleast an hour 4-6 times a week to rid themselves of toxins. A little exploring might be necessary. Again, the bottom line is to find what works for you both physically and emotionally. You want to *want* to exercise. You want to feel good. I tried straight cardio, like running (6 miles), but then I wasn't as tight and trim as when I lifted my heavy weights (and I hurt my hip). When I tried focusing on just the weights, I found that they really helped keep me toned and tight, and that I really didn't bulk *all over* like many people say, but did bulk more in my thigh than I liked. However, my upper body stayed nice and small and tight with it, so I explored some more to see if I could find something good for both.

After lots of searching, experimenting, and input from my fiancé, (with his highly detailed eye) I have found that I don't need anything heavier than 3-pound weights, and I don't need a gym membership. That's the best and most affordable part. I get a serious sweat as long as I find videos (from the $9-$10 rack in Walmart) that run for about an hour, and combine cardio with those light weights by using a lot of my lower body and larger muscle groups to create the cardio effect. I also find I am happiest when doing these or walking. I love having a pool of sweat running off me because I know how much "junk" it is taking with it. I walk whenever possible, but it's the sweat and the blood-flow that really help me to get the toxins out or in a position to be flushed out. These also happen to be what I enjoy doing most, so that just makes me happier and more eager to exercise.

The other benefit I have found from my system (particularly when I think back to a time when I was not in a relationship) is that these workouts also allow me to workout daily, and eliminate the need for me to leave the house for the gym. I can be home with my children, and whether I workout after they are asleep or while they are awake, I have flexibility, now in both my schedule and muscles, and this again has helped me to adapt my healthy lifestyle to my needs and schedule. All I need is a small section of space for me, an art project for the kids, and I am good to go.

Significant others...it doesn't hurt to be as supportive as my fiancé is in helping to make exercise a daily routine. Cooperation and support are key in making exercise part of your regular routine and maintaining a healthy relationship. While my fiancé and I love to work out together, and do as much as we can together, we also recognize that sometimes it is necessary to take turns watching the kids so that we both get our workout in every day. This is a classic illustration of how health begets health. This is also a prime example of how one needs to adapt a system to fit schedules and lifestyles. We have also found that this kind of cooperation and support helps maintain a happy healthy relationship, which also helps to maintain a healthy mind. Well, as long as I continue to ignore the fact that it takes me twice as much work to get the same results he does! Alas, ladies, this is just our design, so enlist as much help from your "other-halves" as you can. They'll appreciate the effort you're making.

A healthy mind is something we'll discuss further when we discuss our other big topics. In the meantime, here are some other ideas for quality exercise routines for those of you who enjoy other forms of exercise:

- Inversions-When I first heard of these, I didn't exactly consider it exercise, but now I do, after learning of and understanding the benefits. I'm sure many of you have heard of these, but for those of you who haven't, they are, literally, as they sound. You are inverting your body. That's right, think Batman. Get upside-down. Hang from a bar, get head-stander, or, use the more commonly known inversion table. Inversions work because they reverse the negative effects of gravity, or just even things out by pulling in the other direction, however you want to think of it. You only need a couple of minutes on your head, but can do whatever you are comfortable with. They also improve the functioning of the lymphatic system, reduce stress, and nourish the brain with an increase in blood flow. Hmmm…can I get about thirty of those for my classroom?

- Yoga-We all know why and how yoga helps. Flexibility, strength-training, and cardio work are important for all of us. Did you know, though, that it also helps to increase the life force? The ancient poses utilized by yoga were actually designed for that purpose. Pretty cool stuff, huh?

- Walking-Honestly, unless you got caught in a hail storm, have you ever NOT felt better after walking? Or felt more depressed? Here's the bottom line: the brain needs oxygen and humans need nature. Go outside and walk, and you accomplish both. You will most likely also find that you sleep better, and we all know that being rested is an important part of being healthy. See how this is all inter-connected, and why we say just trying one thing will lead to more?

- Trampolining-Remember how much fun you had as a kid? There was probably a reason for that, and it is so much less harsh on the body than many other forms of exercise. Don't worry, you don't have to put a huge one in the back yard and go out in the snow. You can purchase small ones, complete with resistance bands, meters, and a DVD workout for under $50. This is great because it also improves lymphatic function, relieves stress, and tones internal organs. Boy, did I laugh picturing that last part, but in this case toning simply means detoxing them and strengthening the connective tissues within the organs themselves. Come on, some of you had visions of your kidney lifting a weight!

Many people are concerned about what happens if they get injured during exercise, and I have experienced minor setbacks due to "over-doing" things as well. Since we are all built differently, "over-doing it" can mean many different things for all of us. I have learned that you can work your way up to an hour of sweat if you aren't there yet, or you can actually just do movement without weights until you feel you can start adding a little resistance. I have also learned to be very careful of my form when I work out, and to maybe move a little slower if it is necessary to help me maintain my form, and therefore protect my muscles, tendons, ligaments, etc. Believe me, it won't set you back. If anything, it gets me added benefit and more sweat from my workout because I am using my muscles more effectively.

Let's say, however, that I do "over-do it" a little, and need to heal and/or repair. Let me start by telling you what I DON"T do in order to get back into tip-top shape, since I want to leave you remembering what TO DO.

In the case that I "over-do it" or get "injured," I **don't**:

- Use creams full of chemicals that are supposed to heal aches and pains. I don't want my body absorbing all of that. (If you wouldn't eat it, don't put it on your skin).

- Take pain-killers, whether they are over-the-counter or prescription. I don't want to put the extra burden of filtering all the toxins on my liver, and I don't want to mask pain that I should probably be feeling so that I don't push something to the point of injury.

- Stop the movement or using that body part all-together! I do take it easier, but I don't want to risk hurting another body part by compensating or having that part seize up on me so that I can't use it at all.

I **do**: (reactive)

- Use natural creams and solvents such as arnica cream or DMSO. My patellar tendon wouldn't be able to keep up with me if I didn't have DMSO to put on it.
- Use ice or heat packs, depending on what the healing need is.

I **do**: (proactive)

- Receive regular chiropractic adjustments. After all, the odds of injuring myself are much greater if I am already out of alignment. (You keep your tires on your car balanced, don't you!) I also don't want my muscles to be tightened up from trying to hold my bones in place.
- Receive occasional acupuncture treatments. I want to keep my muscles loose so they don't tighten and pull my bones out of place, or to remain tight and not allow my bones to be put back in place.
- Remain on a regular detoxification program so that I can perform my workout efficiently and at full strength to avoid injury.

The Next Steps

So, you have now been presented with the basics. We hope that you have been able to find something(s) that you will find manageable and adaptable to your lifestyle. Nothing makes us happier than seeing the people we are trying to help succeed! Now that you have some of the basics, what can you do about all of the factors that may still be facing you? The answer is by controlling the things that you can control. There may be times when you need to ingest or be exposed to something that isn't good for you, or is toxic, but if you do what you can every day to minimize toxicity, those few instances will have significantly less impact on you. We have so many more suggestions and experiences to share with you that have helped us to enhance our healthy life style. Here's what you can do to continue on a healthy path:

- Continue eating as much organic food as you can.
- Continue to avoid white sugar, high fructose corn syrup, and all the other "foods" listed that you should avoid.
- Check your food labels! Beware of terms like "spices," "colorings," and "flavors." These are just code words for "chemicals." Further, "all natural" does not necessarily mean "organic." Even white sugar can legally be called natural. Sometimes I check labels on all natural products and find that the majority of the ingredients are organic, so don't rule them out either. The inconsistency is due to a variety of legislation about what can be printed on labels, which is why overall labels can be misleading, so the best thing to do is read carefully.

- Be aware of your water. If you have a well, congratulations. If your water is from a source that contains chlorine, fluoride, etc., you will want to make sure it is filtered or buy bottled water. We certainly don't promote polluting the environment with bottles of water, so be sure to recycle your bottles. We buy gallon jugs of distilled water for cooking, etc., and Walmart will actually refill those jugs for us for less then it costs to buy a new jug. Ideally, buy a filter for your drinking water AND for your shower as well! Remember, your skin absorbs everything!

- Use only natural soaps, sunscreens, lotions, moisturizers, facial cleansers, etc. Since your skin absorbs everything, remember the rule? And, by the way, the sun doesn't cause cancer. If we have no toxins in our bodies from food, etc., and no chemicals in our skin *from sunscreen*, the sun's rays have nothing to interact with. Most health food stores have natural sunscreens available as well. (Which leads me to my next bullet).

- Get plenty of sunshine! (But don't burn). You can wear long sleeves, hats, etc. to avoid this. Your body NEEDS the sun. It produces essential vitamin D, makes you feel wonderful, and combats depression.

- Get enough sleep. 10 P.M. to 6 A.M. is ideal, but even I can't be guaranteed of that every night. That makes it even more crucial that I follow all of these other healthy recommendations we've given to help give me energy and to function efficiently. However, it is important to try to get enough sleep. Your body releases important healing hormones between 10 P.M. and 2 A.M. We've already established that your body cleanses itself at night, and, finally, I'm sure you've already heard that research shows that people who get enough sleep at night are less likely to be overweight.

- Use a cell phone protector and protect yourself against electromagnetic waves from TV's and other devices. You can find products for this at www.ependantdeal.com.

- Use non-toxic cleaners, hand soaps, etc. These have become very widely available. If you aren't sure if it is toxic or not, check the label. Look for products that say they are plant-based or biodegradable. Even Walmart is now carrying many of these products.

- Re-think your laundry system. Believe it or not, safe laundry detergent is good for more than just the environment. Chemicals from them are left in your clothes, and therefore on your skin, so, again, buy products for the laundry that are plant-based and biodegradable. Also, try to wash new clothes before you wear them. There are a myriad of chemicals on them from factories, shipping, etc.

- Think about what you are breathing in. Most candles, air fresheners, and other things that "smell nice" really are full of chemicals that we breathe in when they burn. We all love it when our house smells nice, so use essential oils, or look for candles that are all-natural. They are becoming more readily available.

- Be choosy in medical/dental care. Do you need an antibiotic, or can you get yourself healthy through the use of exercise, **silverhydrosol, zeolytes**, safe and natural supplements, and good eating habits? Opt for composite fillings at the dentist. We do not need to be putting extra heavy metals in our bodies if at all possible. I also politely say, "No thanks." to the fluoride treatments my dentist always offers to my kids. Of course I get the "she must be a bad parent" looks, but I feel it is easier to deal with tooth issues than it is the issues with their thyroids the fluoride treatments will cause. And, by the way…my kids are 6 and 10, and have never had a cavity.

- Avoid fast food chains, as many add chemicals and non-food items to their food.

- Avoid GMO's…genetically modified organisms and processed foods. Many "disorders" manifesting themselves in children that are being diagnosed and treated with medications, such as ADD, are simply corrected by eliminating processed food from the diet.

- Shop for natural beauty products. Organic make-up is available in many health food stores and on-line. In addition, nail polishes and polish removers are highly toxic. Chemicals and products are absorbed through nails and into the body, so any acrylic, polish, removers, etc. that are used on nails will cause chemicals and toxins to be absorbed into the body.

- Limit the use of prescription and non-prescription drugs. If I get a headache, I find it is usually because I have not hydrated properly for the day, I have a build-up of toxins in me, or my neck is out of alignment, and needs to be adjusted by a chiropractor. So, why would I add more toxins when I already have too much?

- Use digestive aids such as apple cider vinegar. This can be in liquid or pill form. We purchase the pills very inexpensively at www.swansonvitamins.com.

This is how you keep it healthy. Here's how you keep it simple and real: focus on one thing at a time; figure out what your needs are; relax and adapt; don't beat yourself up. This can take a little time, but if you set reasonable goals you will find what you need and accomplish what you want.

So, why couldn't I ditch that size 10 until now? Did I mention that diet has a larger impact on weight than exercise? With that clue, hopefully you have figured out the answer to that question. I was eating processed food that was full of all kinds of things my body could not process, my liver was not "firing on all cylinders," and I was storing toxins in fat cells that I certainly did not need. Exercise can't fix everything. Is wearing my size 2 / 4 about vanity? No. It's about being healthy, and not giving any genetic predispositions to diseases the tools they need to get me later in life. It's about being able to be healthy so I can enjoy an active retirement with my fiancé. Finally, it's about being healthy so I can be *there for* my children and grandchildren and not a *burden on* them. Clearly, what you now see on the outside is somewhat reflective of what's changed on the inside…physically, anyway.

THE MIND

As with any endeavor, it is imperative to be in the right state of mind to ensure success. For some of you, this may be where you feel you need to start. I can certainly understand the need to be able to be clear and focused before trying to sort through all the information that is presented to us. How do you know that you have made the right decisions? Certainly knowing you are in a clear frame of mind helps to ensure that we are making the right decisions. However, I knew that I needed the boost from my physical being to help me to focus on this next step: the mind.

While the mind can be plagued by any number of toxicity issues, perhaps the issue that runs the most rampant among Americans is depression. It has become a virtual epidemic, and what is the solution most often presented to those suffering from depression? Anti-depressants- which, by the way, lose efficacy over time, or else we wouldn't constantly be viewing commercials about additional anti-depressants that are intended to help our initially prescribed anti-depressants work better. If this doesn't ring a bell with you, it is probably because the list of possible negative side effects the commercial presents is actually longer than the benefits the medication offers and you missed the advertisement, so don't feel bad. The anti-depressant charade is really just a vicious cycle that we all fall into, as the prescriptions toxify us further, and therefore actually augment our depression issues. How can one possibly function clearly enough when his mind is muddled by toxins that prevent him from being able to sort through information and make the right health decisions?

I stated earlier that detoxification would be the common denominator in this formula of piecing together a healthy lifestyle. Just as we need to detoxify the body, we need to "detoxify" the mind. Because the three focal points we are addressing in this book are so closely intertwined, "detoxifying"" the mind will also require some detoxification of the body, and is therefore where understanding concepts and not just products becomes essential. We already addressed two of the issues, and therefore, solutions to the problem: *lack of nutrition, and lack of exercise.* These are key components in detoxifying both the body and the mind.

Some other every-day, simple solutions to helping us all "get a grip" include simple activities anyone can do, as well as adding a few supplements to your diet. Whenever you're feeling a little "down," try these natural pick-me-ups:

- Take a daily walk outdoors while looking into the distance.
- Get plenty of sunshine or take vitamin D3 if you live somewhere hit hard by cold winter months with not enough sunshine.

- Consume omega-3 fatty acids via fish oil, flax oil, or coconut oil.
- Get some sort of exercise- oxygen does wonders for the brain.
- Be outside in nature. It's been proven that human beings need to have contact with nature.

While we also try to make activities such as these a part of our daily lifestyle, there are a variety of other techniques we can use to keep us healthy, both physically and mentally. We think they are all great techniques, but you may want to figure out what your greatest need is, and find the technique that will target that need. Try one or try them all- whatever works for you. They all work well for us. Being in a healthy state of mind is just as important as being physically healthy, but, I'll admit, can sometimes be more difficult to maintain. We have also tried maintaining clarity and health for the mind with the following techniques:

Visualization- The concept of visualization is an important component of mental health because of the potential positive impact it can have on the body's nervous system. Most of us are consistently functioning in a state in which the sympathetic nervous system is dominant. This part of the nervous system is triggered by stress and/or fear, which produces toxins in the body. The technique of visualization can help activate the parasympathetic nervous system. This system is responsible for triggering the release of "happy" hormones that help us feel balanced and calm, such as serotonin. It also regulates breathing and lowers heart-rate and blood-pressure. The list goes on- it stimulates digestion and elimination, and doesn't regularity make us all happy?

So, what do you want to visualize? Think of your most important goals, dreams, or desires. You can attain them if you can get yourself very clear about what it is that you truly want. It is important to not have any doubts about your achievement of those goals and to picture them very clearly- hence the term "visualization." If it helps, get pictures of what you want so that you can look at them often. While some of these desires may be very individual and specific to you, other desires are felt by more people than just you- your significant other, or children, perhaps. When we run into that issue, my fiancé and I make sure to discuss very clearly with each other exactly what we want to visualize, so that our concepts are not conflicting. Visualize your goals. Aren't we all happier when we get what we want? And, remember, the universe doesn't understand "not," or "don't." So, focus on what you WANT, rather than what you don't want. For instance, I will visualize *lower gas prices* instead of gas prices not being so high. Maybe if we all did that together...

Meditation-The technique of meditation works very similarly to visualization. The body experiences many of the same benefits. In addition, 20 minutes of deep meditation is equivalent to 2-3 hours of REM sleep! When one enters a state of meditation, the mind enters the alpha state, which is a state that facilitates attracting desires to your life, allows super-learning to occur, and is one of the brainwave states that allows physical healing to take place. It is well-known that those who meditate lead happier and healthier lives, probably because they more easily attract the things that they want into their lives. If you feel like you live life under constant stress, meditation is a great place to start to reduce the stress and ultimately to live a healthier life. If you are having trouble visualizing, you may want to start here, as it may help you to become more clear about what you want, resulting in more effective visualization. If you feel this is too difficult for you, it is possible to purchase CD's that will assist in achieving the meditation state.

Positive thought-This is more powerful than we realize. We reap what we sow, right? So, sow positive thoughts, and reap more positive! Besides, negativity is both mentally and physically draining…it takes more muscles to frown than to smile.

The power of sound-What the **heck** does this have to do with your health? Lots. For years those living in the eastern part of the world have known of and reaped the health benefits of sound. We in the western world are slowly catching up. We've already discussed the fact that we are all happier when we get what we want. We can use the power of sound to further attract the things we want most from the universe. We are also finally beginning to understand that using sound can have positive health benefits. (Remember how good we feel when we get what we want!) One can utilize different sounds to create different results. For example, Dr. Wayne Dyer introduced a self-help CD series entitled *The Secrets to Manifesting Your Destiny* approximately 12 years ago. The focal point of this series was a meditation centering on the sound "AAAAHHHH." As in, "open up and say, "ahhh." Chanting this sound repeatedly while visualizing your deepest desires, such as good health, wealth, success, relationships, finding your car keys, or anything else that may be a dire need opens you to the universe so that the universe may deliver to you, unhindered, what it is that you wanted. "Aaahhh" is the sound of creation, present in every language's term for God or Creator. For example, "Jehovah," "Allah," and even the 'o' in God sounds like "aaahhh." Therefore, by focusing on your desire and chanting this sound repeatedly, you are literally engaging in the process of creation! So, create what you want, for goodness sake!

There are many other practical sounds that we can use to manifest any desire in life, such as the sound, "shreem." This will bring about wealth and material possession when chanted over and over daily. Feeling happier already, aren't you? Especially since now you can definitely afford the organic food your body so desperately needs! The sound "brzee" will bring the same. We spoke earlier of the benefits of remaining positive, and the following sounds can be used to facilitate that process. For example, to help remove all negativity from your life, including debts, litigations, illnesses, etc., speak or write each syllable of the sound "sa-ra-va-na-ba-va-ya" repeatedly.

I'm sure you are wondering how this can possibly work. Ever hear the expression, "Like attracts like?" Well, this is essentially what you are doing with the sounds. You send out the vibration of what you want to the universe, (like) and the universe sends the same vibration back (attracts like). A simpler way to think of it might be like an echo. Here in the Catskill Mountains, we are experts on this. Throw out a sound, and it comes right back. If our mountains were our universe, then what we yell out will be our desires, and it all comes back to us!

For more detailed explanations and more life-enhancing sound frequencies, see Dr. Baskaran Pillai's website www.pathofmiracles.com.

Any guesses about what we love most about these methods? In case you didn't notice…they don't cost a penny! (And they're a lot more pleasurable than taking castor oil).

DEALING WITH KARMA AND INHERITED DISORDER

*N*ow that we have you feeling great physically, and have opened your body and your mind to some really funky stuff, check this out! Ever hear the expression about karma? You know, the one that ends with a bad word? Well, unfortunately for most of us, it's true. But, fortunately, we can create our own good karma as well, and, equally as fortunately, there are ways of detoxifying ourselves of old, bad, and even inherited karma (which is the majority of our karma). We may need to think a little bit more metaphorically here, but you will see how we are all in some way, shape, or form "polluted" by karma and any other disorders passed to us genetically. See, toxicity really is the number one problem affecting all of our lives. Tackling this area of our lives helps us to live healthier, obviously, by helping to minimize the impact of our inherited genetic predispositions so that they do not have significant negative effects on our health. So, what did we do to try to detoxify this area of our lives? We utilized the following programs:

The AIM Program-We need to understand that everything is energy. Energy is neither created nor destroyed, so, essentially, all possibilities for our lives, and every factor of our life is right there for us to grab in frequency form. We carry with us many toxic frequencies, whether we were born with them, inherited them from the environment, or created them ourselves. Many of them negatively impact us, thereby significantly lowering our life force. I'm not a science teacher, but I remember this: "For every action, there is an equal and opposite reaction." Not bad for an English teacher! Anyway, maybe this helps to understand the fact that if there is a frequency for literally *everything*, then there is an opposite frequency for *everything*, right? Just about!

The reason that the AIM program helps us to detoxify is that it determines what frequencies we have that are negatively impacting our lives, and makes available to us the frequency or frequencies that we need to counteract the negatives. Thank goodness. The best part is that the only effort we had to make was to take our pictures and mail in the application. For more information on the AIM program visit www.aimprogram.com.

Karmic-erasing sounds-This technique probably does not warrant much further discussion, as we have already explained how sounds work, as well as the benefit of them. Chanting this particular sound-ma-ka-ral- si (she)-va-ya-na-ma- erases layer upon layer of inherited karma. Therefore, it must be done repeatedly to continue pulling away at the layers. For all you *Shrek* fans, equate inherited karma with an ogre- it has layers like an onion, and can be just as ugly.

CONCLUSION

We certainly hope that you enjoyed reading about our experiences, and, even better, found some aspects real, manageable, and possibly familiar to your own. Ultimately, we hope that you found something that will work for you that you will be able to fit into your busy daily schedule. There really is no single, best way to go about getting healthy. Think about it: isn't any step you take better than no steps taken? While we can't tell you where or how you necessarily need to start, we can share with you what we found worked best for us and hope that you will find comfort and help in some, or, hopefully, all of our experiences. While the healthiest lifestyle consists of a combination of health in these three areas, we know that starting anywhere will ultimately help you to live and feel better, and will therefore help you to take further steps to a healthier lifestyle. No one is perfect. We "stray" from the path occasionally, especially for our kids, but life is all about balance. Do the best you can and congratulate yourself every step of the way. We certainly will.

In an effort to facilitate your process of getting healthy, we have included some of our favorite resources, although this list is by no means exhaustive. There are many wonderful resources available both on-line and locally. You may have to do a little looking, but it is amazing how you will build more and more connections to other fantastic resources as you create your path to better health.

Helpful, Healthy Resources

Cleanses

- Castor oil-Any drug store (or laxative section for that matter) really, but we've tried several different brands, and not all are as odor and taste-free as they claim to be. Our favorite is in our local Walmart.
- Candida cleanse-The most affordable method we have found for this is using silverhydrosol, which is available at www.helpingamericatogether.com. Another, more pricey, but worthy candida cleanse is the Dr. McCombs cleanse, available at www.mccombsplan.com.
- Whole-body cleanse-While a combination of juicing and castor oil will cleanse the entire body, another cleanse that can be purchased is the Be Pure Cleanse, available at www.nowbepurecleanse.com. At www.hempusa.org, one can purchase micro plant powder, which again is

for the entire body, and helps remove heavy metals and countless other health-damaging toxins.

Supplements

- Vitamins, minerals, dietary, and whole-food supplements-We love www.swansonvitamins.com for our health products. The shipping is quite fast, and we have found the products to be very affordable. They also frequently offer significant discounts on products and shipping. Available at www.hempusa.org are storable organic hemp products, which are packed with complete protein, are highly nutritious, and are easily digestible. They can be added to almost anything (such as smoothies) to supplement our diets. For those of you who love fish oil, or really need to take it, try www.pacificrimshop.com to find really awesome fish oil. Finally, if you want another site to search a variety of products on, try www.321supplements.com or www.herbalremedies.com.

- Immune supports-www.naturerich.net sells a fantastic mineral neutralizer that is loaded with highly-absorbable potassium, magnesium, and calcium. It gives our kids TONS of energy! The good kind, not the bad). It is definitely a must-try. Silverhydrosol and zeolytes, available at www.helpingamericatogether.com also significantly reduce the number of absences from school our children have each winter.

Personal Care Products

- Soaps, lotions, toiletries, etc.- www.herbalremedies has all sorts of wonderful products. One of my favorites is the DMSO- the straight-up version. Some of you may want to order the diluted version, however. Previously mentioned, www.naturerich.com is great for this as well, although the inventory is much more product-specific.

Other Great Sites

- www.ependantdeal.com –This site offers EMR and cell phone protection products as well as water filtration products.

- www.grasslandbeef.com –This site offers organic, grass-fed beef. Remember, nature intended cows to eat grass, not grain! Grass-fed, pasture-raised cows are full of vitamins and minerals for you, which actually creates a need to eat less per meal, as you are provided with more nutrients per serving. This saves both money and calories! It's like having your cake, and eating it too… without the calories.

- www.naturalcures.com –Kevin Trudeau's website is brimming with in-depth, comprehensive details regarding just about any health issue you can think of and the natural cure for it. This is for those who are like my fiancé who love to delve into all kinds of facts, details, research, etc. (This book is for people like me, who like the short version.)

- www.discountjuicers.com – Mentioned previously, this website allows consumers to compare a variety of juicers. While not all brands are available, most are, and my favorite part is the comparison tool. Another great website is www.norwalkjuicers.com.
- www.gerson.org –Dr. Gerson's website, with instructions, and many more resources.
- www.eocinstitute.org –This valuable website is home to a plethora of brain-based and sound therapies, which are available for purchase. The Equisync meditation CD series is one of the phenomenal products available. These CD's facilitate the process of achieving a state of meditation.

Other Suggestions

- Buy local.
- Buy organic-milk especially, although finding a milkman is like finding the pot of gold at the end of the rainbow. Raw milk is best.
- Grow your own veggies-but don't put chemicals on them or use chemical fertilizers!
- Make friends with a farmer-and have him raise beef, chicken, etc. for you.
- If necessary, prioritize your organic raw food items with this list: apples, strawberries, grapes, peaches, nectarines, cherries, pears, potatoes, spinach, lettuce, peppers, celery, and tomatoes.
- Take things one step at a time.
- Be well. Be healthy.

Afterword

*B*eing a very visual learner, I find bulleted lists to be most effective in helping me to "cut to the chase" and to find exactly what I need. I suppose that is a bit of the special education teacher in me as well. Create your own or choose from some of the items we have given you. We discussed the concept of visualization, and in order to make that even more concrete, create your own list or visual. It's like your own personal visualization board. The more you are surrounded by it and look at it, the more that you will manifest the healthy lifestyle that you want to achieve, and it takes discipline (and sometimes some thick skin). Discipline is not always easy, but we must do it if we are to follow through. Some days I need to remind myself that this is not the last piece of cake that will ever be staring me in the face! (While I listen to others whisper about how ridiculous it is that I am going to "pass" this time and watch their eyes roll). This is why is so ultimately important to have a healthy mind as well. Just as with anything, giving a little initial effort, especially in the discipline arena, will reap you significant benefits in the end.

Don't let yourself fall into any mindsets that will "trap" you. Here are some of my favorites: "I want to *live*;" "I already had some junk anyway;" "I can't prevent toxins 100% of the time anyway;" etc. My response to the first is, "So do I." My response to most of the rest of these mindsets is, "Of course, so why wouldn't you at least prevent what you can to prevent an overload." I had to chaperone a very long field trip a few weeks ago, and circumstances dictated that I eat food that was, well, less than organic. However, I knew that I could cleanse, and that at least the junk in it wasn't building up in me the way it was in many of the others, because I didn't have the store of toxins they had to begin with. I manage what I can, so that when I don't have a choice, I am not adding to a bad situation the way that others might be.

ABOUT THE AUTHOR

Stephanie resides in Stamford, New York, a rural town in the scenic Catskill Mountains, and is employed as a high school English teacher in Roxbury, New York. In addition to working and raising a family, she continues to pursue a healthy lifestyle. Further, she continues to work with students, parents, peers, and many others who are curious about her experiences and have a desire to create their own healthy way of living. Stephanie is mother and stepmother to three incredible children, and hopes to again work with her fiancé to publish more books in an effort to reach all those who are looking for simplified ways to be healthy.